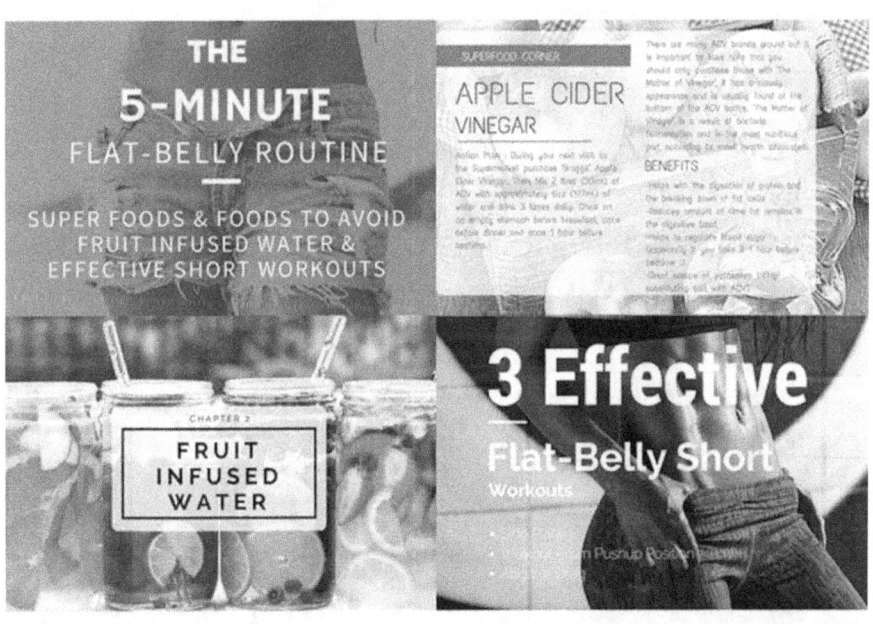
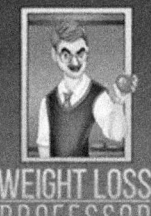

Table of Contents

Introduction

As soon as you've downloaded this book, you've opened yourself up to the many health and fitness benefits of fasting. Fasting is one of the many eating trends that has only taken over the fitness community for the past years, but has been in practice since the ancient times to promote health.

In Defense of Fasting

Fasting is also the cause of many conservatives rolling their eyes in an attempt to express their disgust towards the atrocity of starving one's self just to look and feel good.

Atrocity and starvation - these are emotional and subjective words that put fasting in a very bad light. To put things in the right perspective, allow us to quickly define starvation and take a trip back to history.

Starvation is involuntary. It occurs because there is an absolute absence of food. It's a circumstance the person who is starving cannot control. On the other hand, fasting is a voluntary action. When you choose to fast, you still have control of your circumstance. Therefore, fasting only becomes atrocious when the body is already suffering, but you still choose to continue. This is not what fasting promotes. Apart from weight loss, fasting encourages the formation of an eating pattern that leads to a healthier and fuller life. The fact that there is still "eating" involved with fasting, comparing it to starvation is the real atrocity.

Logically Speaking

There is a reason why the first meal of the day is called breakfast. You've definitely heard about the name's origin back in primary school but for objectivity's sake, let us review what it means. Breakfast means "to break your fast". This is the reason why you normally eat pancakes and eggs to help your body recover from a fasted state that occurred from sleeping. Given this natural occurrence, everyone is, in fact, fasting on a daily basis. But you overslept once and woke up at lunch time one weekend? Then, you are close to following the 16/8 method of intermittent fasting.

History and Medical Use

There is also a reason why doctors would require you to fast before administering a laboratory test, specifically on your blood sample. This is because fasting allows doctors to diagnose the real condition of your health. In fact, fasting was first practiced in the field of medicine during the time of Hippocrates, the Father of Modern Medicine. He even said once "to eat when you are sick, is to feed your illness". Hippocrates sentiment towards fasting has also been supported by his contemporaries - the Greek historian Plutarch and the great philosophers Plato and Aristotle.

The world has also seen fasting advocates in the founding fathers of modern Western medicine, particularly in the father of Toxicology, Philip Parcelsus. He placed fasting in its rightful pedestal by saying "fasting is the greatest remedy, the physician within". Benjamin Franklin was also a proponent of the method. In one of his written works, he said "The best of all medicines is resting and fasting".

Spiritual Roots

Fasting can also be traced in the formation of spiritual habits, specifically in the religion of Islam. Still being observed,

Ramadan promotes fasting among Muslims for four consecutive days. Christians also fast during the observation of Lent, specifically in the Holy Week. Buddhists practice a minimalist lifestyle, letting go of non-essentials that include excessive food.

There are countless facts, studies and testimonials that point towards the efficacy of intermittent fasting. As you go through the various sections of this book, you will discover the myths about intermittent fasting, its real benefits and how you can shift to the eating pattern in just a week.

information is without contract or any type of guarantee assurance.

The trademarks that are used are without any consent, and the publication of the trademark is without permission or backing by the trademark owner. All trademarks and brands within this book are for clarifying purposes only and are the owned by the owners themselves, not affiliated with this document.

Chapter 1 - Before Starting the Switch

Before you start the switch, below are some interesting information about the country's favorite food and beverage establishments.

In the article, *These Are the States with the Most McDonald's*, by *Mark Lieberman* and *Thomas C. Frohlich* of *Time Magazine*, it was reported that there are almost sixteen thousand McDonald's outlets in the country. A 24/7 Wall St. review was also cited in the article, saying states with the most number of McDonald's outlets have the highest rate of obesity in the country. While no one has ever dared to conduct a scientific study to link fast food to weight gain yet, the coincidental outcome of the said review speaks more than just numbers.

Speaking of numbers, take a look at what a Starbucks Vanilla Latte contains:

STARBUCKS VANILLA LATTE

- 250 calories
- 36 grams of carbohydrates
- 34 grams of sugar
- 12 grams of protein
- 6 grams of fat

If you have been asking your friendly barista to top your favorite coffee concoction with the very indulging whipped cream, you are certainly requesting an additional serving of the following:

- 80 calories
- 3 grams of carbohydrates

- 3 grams of sugar

- 1 gram of protein

- 8 grams of fat

What is the point of telling you what seems to be trivial information in respect to intermittent fasting? To breed fear? Badmouth America's favorite fast food and beverage chain? The answer to the last two questions is a resounding NO. The whole point of dishing this information out to you is to become aware of what you have been unhealthily feeding yourself out of habit for so long. This is because keeping these habits will defeat the purpose of changing your dieting pattern. In a later discussion about diets, you will also find out why you should avoid fast food and unhealthy beverages when fasting.

If you are serious about losing weight through intermittent fasting, unhealthy fast food and beverages are the first to get the boot out of your diet, which brings us to the first two pro-tips to starting the dieting pattern change.

PRO- TIP

1. Replace fast food favorites with healthier alternatives. Instead of eating fat- and sodium-induced French fries, try baked sweet potatoes.

2. Change your quick coffee fixes with Café Americano. It is enough to keep you going the rest of the day. At the same time, you are just consuming about 30 calories of it, a gram of sugar, a gram of carbs, and two grams of fat.

   Furthermore, you do not have to give up visiting Starbucks after all, as they serve this brew in most if not in all of their outlets.

A Dieting Pattern

With what you have read so far, you are probably thinking you will be forced to painstakingly follow a specific set of guidelines to complete the switch. While you certainly need to make a few sacrifices during the transition, intermittent fasting is not like any conventional diet plan you know. This is because it is not exactly a diet, but a dieting pattern.

Main Requirement

The truth is intermittent fasting primarily requires the person who wants to undertake it to have an open mind. Reading this now means you have one. Therefore, all you need is to gain more information about the dieting pattern, so you can broaden your current understanding of it, and inspire yourself to form a healthy eating habit.

Learning the Truth

As a beginner, one of the most important parts of the transition is knowing as many facts as possible about the dieting pattern. However, some information you have known to be correct for the longest time may disrupt the transition. The only way to avoid this from happening is to unlearn them as early as now.

Breaking the Breakfast Belief

A popular belief you need to unlearn is *"eating breakfast promotes weight loss"*. Breakfast has always been considered the most important meal of day. It also means "to break your fast", which contradicts with the principle of this dieting pattern - to subject your body into a fasted state.

Some people argue that a full meal in the morning provides the body with the energy it needs for the rest of the day. It also intensifies metabolism, which leads to burning extra fats. Therefore, it does not matter if they splurge on food in the morning, eat some at lunch and skip dinner altogether. They are already losing weight so why would they even punish their bodies just to lose it?

Another belief you would want to unlearn is *"rewarding the body with small portions of food helps in losing more weight"*. Some people follow this principle by rewarding their bodies with minimal portions of their regular meal a number of times a day, usually six times, within a 24-hour period. It has been said that this eating pattern allows the body to maximize its metabolic function, which results to losing weight.

Again, this pattern is stark of a considerable period of fasting. However, advocates of this eating pattern argue that there is no need to force the body to suffer just to shed the extra pounds. Why not reward the body with the nourishment it needs for doing a great job of losing its unnecessary fats?

Settling the Dust

With these two beliefs you need to unlearn, ask yourself these questions:

- What if I am not really hungry, does it mean I have to eat breakfast just to get through the day and lose weight?

- What if I woke up late? Does it mean I already skipped the most important meal of the day?

- Does it mean I am not maximizing the metabolic functions of my body if I do not have the luxury of time just to eat multiple smaller portions of my regular meal?

No! No! and No!

At least with the main principle of intermittent fasting, the answer to these questions is NO. You are probably thinking you have been negating most of the circumstances related to your regular eating habits. Nullifying dieting habits makes this dieting pattern absolutely controversial, but it is also what is making it work. Experts cannot stress enough the importance of saying NO to these eating habits to succeed in this journey.

As you move on with reading this eBook though, you will find more reasons why you need to say YES to intermittent fasting.

Chapter 2 - Understanding the Different Fasting Methods

SAY YES TO THIS!

Skip breakfast or any of your regular meals within a specific period of time.

- It encourages your body to grow and build more muscles.

- It optimizes many bodily functions, particularly your metabolic processes.

- It helps you lose more weight.

Contrary to what other people believe, intermittent fasting is not all about suffering and sacrifices. In fact, it still encourages you to feast on food in a particular part of the day and completely avoid it during the rest. You fast to enhance the body's different functions and you reasonably feast to help it recover. To help you and your doctor or dietitian decide what would best work for you, below are six common fasting methods followed by many intermittent fasting advocates.

Spontaneous Fasting

Among the methods, spontaneous fasting is the easiest and the most convenient to follow. As the name suggests, the method is done spontaneously and mostly at your convenience. This is because you are not following a timed structure as the other methods require.

This method is designed for beginners and people who follow a fixed schedule for other concerns have to prioritize the said schedule.

As a beginner, a medical practitioner may prescribe this method of fasting to get a feel of it and quickly assess your body' reaction to starvation.

You normally start this method on the spot. For example, if you are on the field and cannot find a healthy place to eat out, you can forego eating for at least one or two hours until you find a place where you can eat something healthy.

You can also use the morning rush hour as an opportunity to jumpstart fasting. If you are in a hurry to get to the office on time and avoid traffic, you might as well skip your regular breakfast and head to the office or school right away. It will be much better if you can walk to the office. Keep in mind that fasting and exercising complement each other in terms of shedding those unhealthy fats stored in the body.

PRO TIP

No one ever said you cannot drink water when you are fasting.

Remember to keep your body hydrated when it is in a fasted state. Water will not only help your body burn fats faster, it also refreshes its temperature and helps you deflect false hunger signals sent to your brain.

So, the next time you feel hungry, drink a glass of cold water and drive false hunger pains away.

The Warrior Diet

Popularized by fitness expert and blogger Ori Hofmekler, this is one of the many diet principles that suits the dieting pattern.

The diet principle involved is the Paleo diet. So, if you are a staunch believer of the said principle, you may want to use this method.

With the warrior diet, you are supposed to eat only small portions of raw vegetables and fruits during the day and recover by eating a large meal at night. Since this is a Paleo diet, you need to make sure all foods you eat are organic and unprocessed. Also, remember that you have a 4-hour window at night to eat your Paleo meal.

PRO TIP

It's quite a challenge to find organic food in the grocery. Your best sources of anything organic are small neighborhood farms and your backyard. Try infusing your garden with small fruit and vegetable-bearing plants for your plant-based Paleo diet during the day. For your meat-based Paleo meal, just remember - anything that is mass -produced is definitely not Paleo.

The Warrior Diet

Time of Day	Monday	Tuesday	Wednesday	Thursday	Friday	Saturday	Sunday
Day Meal			Fruit and Vegetables Only				
Night Meal			Paleo meals only between 6 PM to 9PM				

Alternate Fasting

This method is probably the most extreme among the six most popular methods. This method requires you to subject your body to a full fasted state today then eat normally the following day. The day after the next, you go back to a complete fasted state.

Because of its extreme nature, this is not recommended for beginners like you, although there is a version that is less extreme. This version of alternate fasting allows you to eat 500 calories during the non-fasting day.

You can switch to this dieting pattern once your body has completely adjusted to the other methods, but only with the full recommendation of your doctor or dietitian. Otherwise, you may overwhelm your body and disrupt the dieting pattern for good.

Alternate Fasting

Monday	Tuesday	Wednesday	Thursday	Friday	Saturday	Sunday
Fasting Day	Non-Fasting Day	Fasting Day	Non-Fasting Day	Fasting Day	Non-Fasting Day	Fasting Day (The following should follow the pattern. This means tomorrow would be a non-fasting ay

Eat-Stop-Eat Pattern

This intermittent fasting method was invented by Brad Pilon and has been circulating the fitness community for several years now.

Similar to what you may already know about intermittent fasting, the general structure of this method is a full blast fasting for 24 hours for two non-consecutive days.

During the fasting days, you may drink non-caloric beverages, like sugar and dairy-free coffee and tea, but not anything solid. Even fitness experts confess experiencing difficulties keeping up with this structure. Therefore, subjecting yourself into this fasting method requires careful planning and evaluation of your overall fitness. This is to gauge your ability to sustain a fasted-state for a full day after your body has adjusted to a normal dieting structure.

Others recommend gradually increasing your fasting period from fourteen hours to sixteen hours before moving on to the 24-hour fasting window.

Eat-Stop-Eat Pattern

Monday	Tuesday	Wednesday	Thursday	Friday	Saturday	Sunday
Normal Eating Day	Normal Eating Day	Normal Eating Day Last meal should end by 8 PM	Fasting Day from 8PM the previous day to 8PM (24 hours), 12NN (16 hours) or 10AM (14 hours) today	Normal Eating Day	Normal Eating Day Last meal should end by 8 PM	Fasting Day from 8PM the previous day to 8PM (24 hours), 12NN (16 hours) or 10AM (14 hours) today

The Fast Diet

Also known as the 5:2 Diet, the method follows this week-long cycle - you eat normally for five days and dedicate two days for fasting.

Introduced by Dr. Michael Mosley to the fitness community many years ago, the method does not actually promote complete starvation while in the cycle. Women are recommended to consume 500 calories of food on their selected fasting days. You can start your transition using this method and level up once you have practiced self-control.

The Fast Diet

Monday	Tuesday	Wednesday	Thursday	Friday	Saturday	Sunday
Fasting Day 500 calories of food	Normal Eating Day	Normal Eating Day	Fasting Day 500 calories of food	Normal Eating Day	Normal Eating Day	Normal Eating Day

16/8 Fasting

The most popular among the fasting methods, the 16/8 fasting requires you to remember the two main components that define its structure – the fasting period of 16 hours and the eating window of 8 hours.

In this method, also known as the Leangain Protocol, every day is a fasting day. The only leeway you will have is fitting a maximum of three meals within the eight-hour eating window.

Women may also adjust the fasting period to 14 to 15 hours to maintain the momentum and help their body adjust to the very long period of fasting.

16/18/ Leangain Protocol

Component	Monday	Tuesday	Wednesday	Thursday	Friday	Saturday	Sunday
Fasting Period	12 MN– 12 NN (including 8PM to 12 MN of the previous day						
Eating Window	12 NN – 8PM Note: Fit a maximum of three meals between these times.						

Chapter 3 - The Science behind Intermittent Fasting

Intermittent fasting is not a stranger to the skepticism of many people, especially those who follow an entirely different method of dieting. Even you may still have doubts about its credibility as an effective weight loss therapy.

It is true that the information you have been presented so far is not yet sufficient to encourage you to make the switch. This is the reason why in this section, we are presenting you science-based explanations that will further inspire you to make that important decision about changing your dieting pattern.

It all begins with the same argument presented in the first chapter - shall you eat or skip breakfast?

Eating Breakfast = Minimal Weight Loss

If you skip breakfast, you tend to eat as much food as you can at lunch and at dinner, allowing your body to lose steady amount of fats over time. This happens because there is still a deficit in your recommended daily calorie intake to maintain weight. While this already sounds promising, it does not really optimize the body's weight loss functions.

But why is this so?

Timing is Key

Apart from the fact that not all calories are created the same, your body also reacts differently towards calorie intake at a given time of the day. In a study presented by the *International Journal of Obesity*, it was revealed that eating late can influence weight loss. The study recommends incorporating the timing of food consumption with the conventional ways of ensuring weight loss – distributing macronutrients and counting calorie intake.

This research alone, along with a number of similar scientific studies, is enough to say timing is an important consideration you make to maximize the body's fat burning functions.

PROOF THAT CALORIES ARE NOT CREATED THE SAME

100 grams of bacon has 541 calories while the same amount of broccoli would only have 34 calories. Even if it is possible for you to consume almost two kilograms of broccoli in one sitting (just to equal the calorie-content of probably 3-5 strips of bacon), you are not eating any fat at all. On the other hand, those bacon strips contain a total of 42 grams of fat.

What your Body Does when you Eat and Don't Eat Food?

Normally, your body processes food between six to eight hours. During these hours, it takes advantage of the food it is processing and turns it into an energy source. When this happens, fats already stored in your body are literally ignored and remain unprocessed. The body bypassing stored fats become more intense when it finds more carbs and sugar to use as fuel and release into the bloodstream.

When your body is in a fasted state, it obviously does not have any food to source its energy from. Therefore, it makes do with stored body fats, burns and turns them into your much needed energy. Over time, you lose unwanted fats that are pulling your weight down.

This body processing food phenomenon is the reason behind the long fasting windows in the various methods discussed in the previous chapter.

Fasting and Exercising = Optimal Weight Loss

The body burning fats is further optimized with a prescribed workout program. When you exercise, you need more energy to keep up and finish it. Given that you are fasting at the time you are working out, your body will help itself recover from the activity by burning whatever source it has into energy. Because your stomach is empty of food, your body uses stored fats. If you combine fasting and exercising, just imagine how much weight you will be losing over time.

Fasting Spurs Insulin Sensitivity

Intermittent fasting allows the body to react accordingly with the food it has to process and the insulin it is has to produce. If your body is sensitive to insulin, it is more likely to use the food you ate more efficiently, leading to weight loss and even muscle buildup.

When you eat any sugar or carb-rich food, the body processes and turns it into glucose, which is then released into the bloodstream for your cells to use as energy. Your pancreas then releases insulin to help the cells and your muscle tissues absorb glucose. When you have less sugar in your blood, the less insulin it tends to release. This is when you become insulin sensitive. But how does this relate to weight loss and muscle buildup?

You tend to lose weight because your body's sensitivity to insulin prepares your cells to absorb and convert glucose into energy quickly, rather than store them as fats. The same goes with your muscle tissues. When the muscles absorb glucose along with other nutrients, protein synthesis happens within, resulting to muscle growth and buildup.

Fasting and Glycogen

Your body stores glycogen in your liver and muscles and uses it as energy when necessary. Even when you are asleep, stored glycogen are being used up by the body. Therefore, when your body is in a fasted state then you start the next day skipping your meal and working out, you are further emptying your body of glycogen. This also results to increasing your body's sensitivity to insulin, but more importantly, it causes your body to make up for the loss as soon as you eat later in the day. Instead of storing the food it processed as fats, the body converts calories into glycogen and immediately stores them as energy.

To see the difference more clearly, just imagine how your body processes food on a regular day. Your body is not in a fasted state and its sensitivity to insulin is at a normal level. Since the body has processed enough food during breakfast and already stored food components as glycogen, the next time you eat, the food it will process will be stored as fats.

On the other hand, your body in a fasted state does not have a choice but to process stored fats and turn them into energy as soon as possible. If this occurs frequently in an intermittent basis over time, then it is not impossible to shed as much pounds as you need.

> ## GLUCOSE VS. GLYCOGEN
>
> Glucose is a simple sugar while the other is complex. When there is an excess of simple sugar in your body, they are processed and stored in the liver as glycogen.

Fasting and Autophagy

In relation to a fasted body assisting cells in the absorption of essential food components from the bloodstream, fasting also encourages their auto repair through the physiological process known as autophagy. Autophagy occurs when your cells remove the buildup of old and non-functional proteins from their structures. This was proven in a study conducted by the *Scripps Research Institute* in 2010. With frequent autophagy through fasting, you can expect more efficient cellular functions and leaner muscles.

Fasting and Metabolism

A primary factor in weight loss therapies, metabolism is considerably affected when you subject your body to a fasted state. Various studies, particularly the study conducted by the Queens Medical Center in Nottingham, UK, revealed that starvation may increase metabolic rate between 3.6 to 14%. The increase in metabolic rate is supported mainly by the release of hormones in the body, specifically norepinephrine or noradrenaline.

Also known as stress hormone, norepinephrine aids in releasing more sugar in the body so muscles will have something to feed on, especially when you are hungry or consciously starving yourself.

Effect on Obesity

A study conducted by the University of Illinois revealed intermittent calorie restriction done within three to twelve weeks by obese individuals resulted to 4 to 8% of weight loss, while daily calorie restriction within the same period allowed subjects to lose 5 to 8 % of their weight. While the two study methods showed almost similar results, it also revealed that intermittent calorie intake restriction caused 11 to 16% of lean mass loss compared to daily calorie restriction's 10 to 20%. This suggests intermittent fasting does not only encourage weight loss, but also allows you to keep lean muscles over time.

Chapter 4 – Health and Fitness Benefits of Intermittent Fasting

Apart from its weight loss benefit, intermittent fasting provides a number of health and fitness benefits to people following any of the dieting pattern's most popular methods. These benefits are either results of losing unhealthy body weight or the healthy side effects of fasting itself.

Lowering the Risks of Diabetes

As you may already know, the production of insulin is affected when you subject your body to a fasted state. When insulin is efficiently released to the body, it lowers your blood sugar level because glucose is properly distributed to the cell tissues for absorption. As a result, unwanted sugar components are removed from your bloodstream, therefore lowering your risk of developing type 2 diabetes.

In a clinical study featured in Translational Research: The Journal of Laboratory and Clinical Fasting, intermittent calorie restriction among human subjects for three days within a week revealed a reduction in the subjects' blood sugar levels (3 to 6%) and an increase in their fasting insulin levels (20-31%).

Anti-inflammatory

Another study conducted by experts of Maltepe University School of Medicine located in Istanbul, Turkey revealed the anti-inflammatory effects of intermittent fasting. In the study, twenty women were subjected to a 12-hour daily food and beverage intake for thirty days, which is similar to what Muslims do when observing Ramadan. Blood samples of the subjects showed a decrease and improvement in the following components:

C-reactive protein

Produced by the liver, this substance is a main inflammatory indicator. When there is an ongoing inflammation in the body, the level of C-reactive protein in the body increases. Therefore, a lower or a decreased level of this substance is a healthy body indication.

Homocysteine

This is an amino acid that naturally occurs in the body to help methionine and cysteine synthesize proteins. As good as its function sounds, high levels of homocysteine show possible inflammation in essential parts of the cardiovascular system. Consequently, a low level of this amino acid could indicate a healthy heart.

Total Cholesterol (TC)/High Density Lipoprotein (HDL)ratio

This ratio indicates that the closer the HDL level is with the TC, the better your health condition is. This is because HDL is considered the good cholesterol, as opposed to LDL (low density lipoprotein) cholesterol, which forms part of the TC in this ratio.

Reduced Risk of Hypertension

To support the previous claim even further, another study conducted by the University of Illinois revealed that alternate fasting reduces blood triglycerides and LDL cholesterol. In the study, 12 women were administered with only 25% of their daily calorie needs on their fasting days within the 10-week trial period. The study resulted to the subjects reducing their triglyceride and LDL cholesterol levels by 6% and 10%, respectively.

Possible Anti-Cancer Effects

The results of a study conducted by the Norris Cancer Center, University of Southern California revealed differential stress sensitization of cancer cells, including breast cancer cells, occur with starvation or fasting. Since cancer cells feed on nutrients as well, a fasted state inhibits their growth and leads to their apoptosis or death.

Brain Health

Intermittent fasting also promotes brain health. This has been proven in numerous scientific studies, particularly the research conducted by the John Hopkins University School of Medicine in Baltimore, Maryland. The study showed reducing the frequency of meals could increase the production of brain-derived neurotrophic factor (BDNF), a brain hormone which helps the neurons to resist degeneration and dysfunction.

A further study by National Institute on Aging, Intramural Research Program in Baltimore, Maryland supported the claim made by educational institution, adding that fasting can reduce the risks of cognitive dysfunction or ailments like Alzheimer's disease.

Anti-aging Factor

Lastly, another study by the National Institute on Aging showed that the fasting of rats increased their lifespan by 36% to 83%. While a similar study is yet to be conducted on humans to prove intermittent fasting's anti-aging side effects, it has already shown a lot of promise. After all, constant exposure to food, especially unhealthy ones, is known to be the cause of many human diseases.

Chapter 5 - Women and Intermittent Fasting

While intermittent fasting provides health and fitness benefits, women must take additional precautions before switching to the diet. This is because women possess an entirely different and sensitive physiological structure. Obviously, if you are underweight or if you have a history of any of the two eating disorders (anorexia nervosa and bulimia nervosa), you must not start fasting until you receive both a verbal and a written permission from your physician.

General Side Effects

Although no scientific study has been conducted on human females yet, the result of a study conducted by the National Institute of Aging on female rats revealed infertility, emaciation and even masculinization among the subjects. These three occurred after being exposed to a restricted food intake.

Disrupted Cycle

There are also reports that women who undergo intermittent fasting disrupted their normal menstrual cycle, a condition known as amenorrhea. These reports are largely supported by how female hormones react towards fasting, which is apparently extreme.

In females, the hypothalamus and the pituitary gland release gonadotropin releasing hormone (GnRH); as well as follicular stimulating and luteinizing hormones, respectively. These hormones trigger the release of progesterone and estrogen from the ovaries after thirty days from the previous menstruation. As you may already know, both hormones released from the female gonads support ovulation and pregnancy.

Since these female hormones are extremely sensitive to calorie intake, intermittent fasting can affect their timely release. This is also the reason why intermittent fasting is prohibited when you are trying to conceive a baby or currently pregnant.

A Note to Women

Therefore, you must undergo a full medical check-up before proceeding with the dieting pattern switch. For your reference, here are some health conditions and circumstances your doctor should evaluate prior to fasting:

- Weight, especially if you are underweight
- Irregularities in blood sugar level
- Abnormal blood pressure
- Under any regular medication
- Eating disorder
- Irregular menstrual cycle
- Wanting to be pregnant or currently pregnant
- Breastfeeding

Safety First

If you will analyze everything that has been discussed in this section, it seems intermittent fasting largely affects your body's reproductive system and functions. What if you are not trying to conceive a baby or not expecting to be pregnant soon? What if you have been experiencing irregular menstruation ever since?

Remember there are no exceptions to ensuring your safety until you receive the go signal from your physician.

Chapter 6 - The Weekly Plan

Once you are cleared and your doctor approves of your plan to undergo intermittent fasting, it is time to draft your plan. Of course, you still need to communicate the said plan to your doctor.

Unconscious Fasting

In the past, you have probably and unconsciously followed the spontaneous fasting method. Even at present, you are spontaneously fasting every time you skip your meals because you are not hungry or you are busy doing more important activities. Therefore, following this protocol may not be optimally beneficial as a beginner's fasting method.

The Beginner's Method

Among the remaining five methods, 16/8 is definitely your best bet to outlast the 7-day shifting period. It is also the method that will surely get your doctor's approval. If you'll look closely at the sample schedule for 16/8 fasting method, you are not completely starving yourself in any given day. In fact, it is similar to spontaneous fasting. The only difference is this - you have a daily fasting schedule with the 16/8 method.

Planning Your Week

In the first five days of the transition week, it will be easier to outlast the fasting window. Technically, you'll spend eight hours for sleeping (from 10 PM the night before until 6AM the following day) and another eight hours for working (probably from 9AM to 5PM the next day). Therefore, you'll only have three hours in the morning to possibly feel hungry and two hours in the evening to crave for food.

To work around these hours, you may want to exercise for an hour in the morning and use the remaining time to prepare for work or school. While at work or school, keep yourself busy until lunch time. Lunch time is when you reward yourself with healthy food, and help your body recover after completing the fourteen hours of fasting. Once you are done eating your last meal of the day at home and the clock strikes 8, plan for the next day's activities (1 hour) and prepare to sleep (1 hour).

The most challenging part of the transition period is getting through the weekend. During the weekend, your brain will have more time to remind you of what you have been missing. To avoid this from happening, pre-plan your weekend activities with loved ones. As much as possible, plan activities that will physically and mentally stimulate you. You can play your favorite sports or challenge everyone in the family to a game of Scrabble.

PRO-TIP

Declutter your food pantry and fridge during the weekend. This means you need to dispose unhealthy food items and keep the ones that adhere to the principles of your chosen diet plan. Decluttering does not only encourage simple eating habits. It also promotes simple and organized thinking.

It's been mentioned many times in this e-book that intermittent fasting is not a diet but a dieting pattern. In that case, you must follow a diet that fits and completes the 16/8 method.

Compatible Diet Principles

Three of the most popular diets in the world today are Paleo, Keto and Vegetarian. The following shall give you an idea about what each diet covers and how it fits the dieting pattern.

- Paleo Diet

  This type of diet encourages the consumption of any food, as long as they are not processed and were farmed like they were farmed during the Paleolithic era. Therefore, a Paleo diet would not include grains, mass-produced or factory farmed meat, etc. Since this diet relies on healthy animal fats to provide your much-needed energy, it fits with the main principle of intermittent fasting - use stored fats as energy and lose weight in the process.

- Keto Diet

  Also known as the Ketogenic diet, the name was derived from the word "ketosis". Ketosis occurs when the body burns fat to produce energy. Similar to the Paleo diet, it encourages the consumption of naturally occurring fats from meat. If you haven't tried the diet yet, you may find its principle contradictory to the principles of the other two diets, and what you may know about fats. It promotes natural fats as healthy components of foods and even encourages followers to have as many fatty components included in their daily meals.

- Vegetarian Diet

  This is probably the type of diet you are most familiar with. While the diet has evolved into many different versions (like eating dairy along with vegetables and fruits or purely eating vegetables), it encourages filling the body with fiber instead of carbs. A few servings of vegetables can easily make you feel full. This is because of the natural fiber contained in it. When this happens, you automatically lower the amount of calorie you ingest, forcing the body to process stored fats as energy.

The three diet principles also agree on the following:

1. Fast food and processed food are definitely unhealthy.

2. Carbs and sugar do not promote health and fitness.

Given the similar perspectives of the diets, they all complement the 16/8 intermittent fasting method. In fact, proponents of the three diet types encourage the use of intermittent fasting when transitioning to any of the three diets.

Doctor's Approval

As always, you are highly advised to seek the assistance and approval of a licensed medical expert when incorporating any of the diets with intermittent fasting. Again, safety is still your main priority.

Dealing with Withdrawal

Withdrawal symptoms will occur once you start the shift. To sustain fasting and avoid giving in to the symptoms, refrain from consuming toxic foods, like processed meat, junk food, candies and sweets. Cut toxic habits that intensify the symptoms like smoking and sleeping late.

> **PRO TIP**
>
> Help yourself overcome withdrawal symptoms intensified by bad habits with meditation and yoga. For fifteen minutes daily, sit in a lotus position in a quiet area in the house. Close your eyes then slowly breathe in and out. Meditation does not only lessen the pains of withdrawal, but also helps you break those bad habits in the long run.

Last Meal of the Day Tip

For your last meal of the day, restrict food items with high amounts of sugar. As you may already know, sugar-rich food items promote a condition called sugar rush. A sugar rush will only trigger hunger, which then leads to breaking the fast earlier than actually intended. The same thing goes with high-carb foods as carbohydrates are converted in the body into simple and complex sugars.

Cutting Calorie-Intake

Your doctor may also recommend not cutting your calorie intake during the eating window (12 NN-8PM). This is reasonable as the real benefit of fasting occurs during the fasting window and not during the eating window. As mentioned earlier, this is the time you physically and mentally reward your body with healthy food choices.

Expert Recommendation on Calorie Intake

Conservatively, your recommended daily calorie intake is between 1600 and 2000. According to the United States Department of Agriculture (USDA), you can estimate your daily energy needs by multiplying your weight (in pounds) by 13.

Stick to your calorie intake goal during your eating window. You can only restrict your calorie intake when you are already following the more advanced methods of fasting.

Supplements

Contrary to what others say, supplements do not interrupt the fasting process. In fact, experts recommend taking branched-chain amino acids when you are working out in a fasted state. Just remember to take the supplement during your first meal.

A Realistic View

Lastly, be realistic about your goals. During the transition period, you will not experience an extreme weight loss. It is only during the time when your body has fully adjusted to the regimen can you start seeing a considerable change in your body weight.

Needs vs. Wants

The main purpose of the transition period is to break your eating habits (eating meals at certain times of the day). When the habit has been broken, your body's various functions automatically adopt to your new eating pattern. This is when you will know that your eating lifestyle has changed. You eat because you need to and because you simply want to.

Conclusion

While intermittent fasting requires you to break old habits, unlearn the common knowledge about patterned eating and undergo a comprehensive evaluation of your current health condition, its long-term benefits cannot be discounted.

The benefits of a changed eating pattern brought about by intermittent fasting do not only address the issue of obesity, but also the physiological conditions that put your health at risk - hypertension, diabetes and inflammatory ailments.

The method may have been questioned by many conservatives, but numerous scientific studies have proven its efficacy in addressing the health concerns of those who believe in it.

Moral and Ethical

Intermittent fasting may pose some restrictions to women like you, but these limitations prove that the method remains to be moral and ethical. Just consider its spiritual roots and its adherence to the religious principles of food abstinence (Islam and Christianity) and minimalism (Buddhism).

Flexibility

While intermittent fasting is not designed for everyone, the fact that there are already six methods you can follow means you can still fast based on your current health condition and doctor's recommendation.

Like most of your endeavors, start small and advance when you are ready. As presented in this e-book, begin your transition with the 16/8 method. Combining your instincts and the expert advice of a doctor, level up to more advanced methods, like 5:2 or the alternate day fasting method.

Moreover, intermittent fasting will not interfere with your current diet principle, if you already have one. As long as a medical expert can guarantee your fitness to undertake the method, you will not change the entirety of your food preference. Whether your daily meals are plant-based or meat-based, you can still implement intermittent fasting.

Habit Forming

In reality, any diet or dieting pattern cannot promise considerable results during the early stages of its implementation. However, a successful transition within a week's time can guarantee the formation of a habit.

Timing is definitely the most important component of transitioning to a healthy eating pattern. Start when you are ready, but remember not to break the momentum once you are in the habit.

With a few sacrifices, you'll pull through the challenge and without you noticing it, you are already reaping the benefits of a changed eating lifestyle.

Congratulations for reaching this part of the book. Thank you very much for trusting us to help you begin your journey towards a healthier and fitter lifestyle.

If you may, share what you have learned in this eBook to the people you love the most. As they say, there is nothing more fulfilling than encouraging your loved ones to reap the same benefits you have received from an endeavor such as this.

Finally, if you enjoyed this book, then I'd like to ask you for a favor, would you be kind enough to leave a review for this book on Amazon? It'd be greatly appreciated!

Click here to leave a review for this book on Amazon!

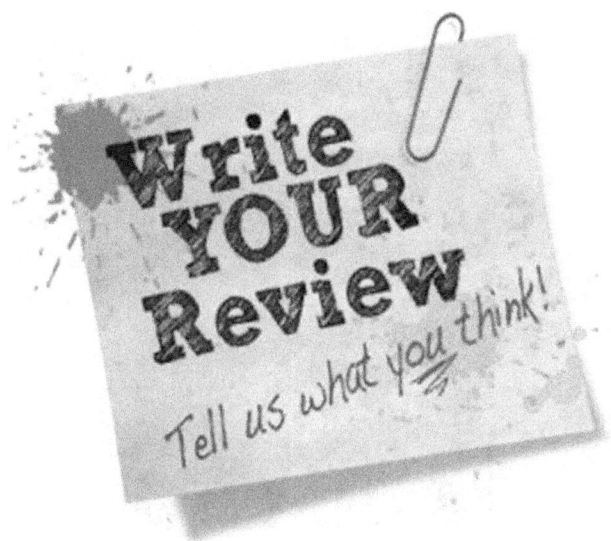

Thank you and good luck!

Preview Of 'The Skinny Asian Chef's Stir-Fry Recipes'

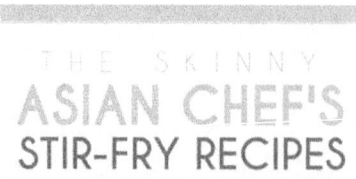

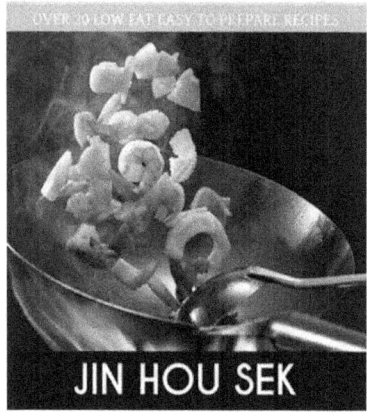

Introduction

This book contains proven steps and strategies on how to stir-fry delicious, healthy, low fat and low carb foods.

Stir-frying is a healthy way of cooking food because it does not heat the vegetables and other nutrient-filled ingredients for too long, and it does not call for the use of a lot of fatty ingredients. By choosing to prepare stir-fried foods regularly, you will easily achieve weight loss without sacrificing your health.

In this book, you will discover the best techniques on how to stir-fry your way to a skinny (but still healthy) body. More importantly, you will learn how to prepare over 25 stir-fry Asian recipes including vegetables, rice, noodles, seafood, poultry, pork and beef.

[Click here to check out the rest of 'The Skinny Asian Chef's Stir-Fry Recipes' on Amazon.](#)

Check Out My Other Books

Below you'll find some of my other popular books that are popular on Amazon and Kindle as well. Simply click on the links below to check them out. Alternatively, you can visit my author page on Amazon to see other works published by me.

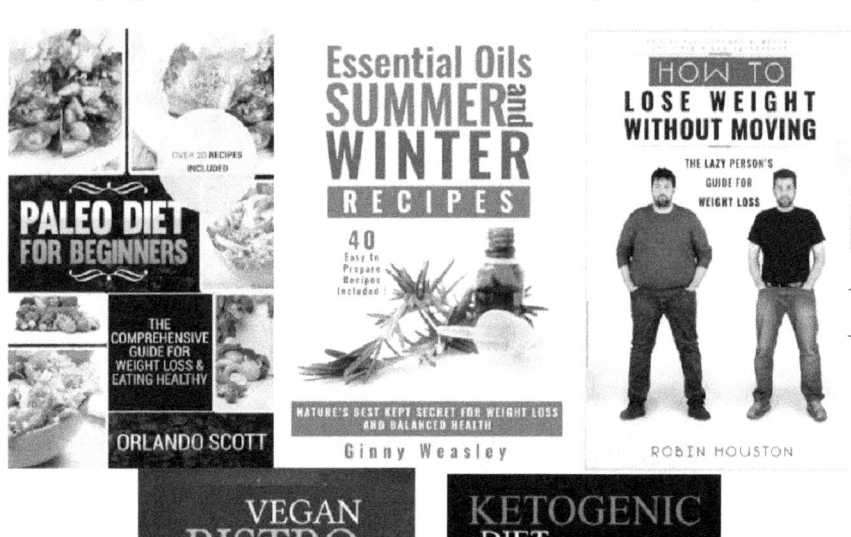

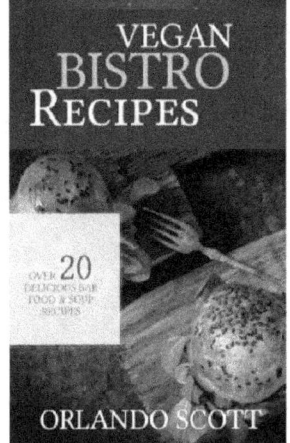

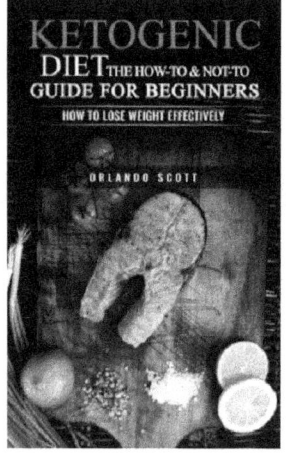

Paleo Diet For Beginners Link

Essential Oils Summer And Winter Recipes Link

How To Lose Weight Without Moving Link

<u>Vegan Bistro Recipes Link</u>

<u>Ketogenic Diet Link</u>

If the links do not work, for whatever reason, you can simply search for these titles on the Amazon website to find them.

www.ingramcontent.com/pod-product-compliance
Lightning Source LLC
Chambersburg PA
CBHW071142280526
45787CB00003B/1370